I0841727

High-Intensity Interval Training (HIIT)

Accelerate Your Fitness Gains

Table of Contents

Chapter 1. Introduction

Embrace a revolutionary approach to fitness that's taking the world by storm! Welcome to our Special Report: High-Intensity Interval Training (HIIT) - Accelerate Your Fitness Gains. Packed to the brim with comprehensive guides, expert advice, and scientific insights, this report details a fitness regime that delivers promising results in less time. Whether you're an accomplished athlete or starting your fitness journey, this special report is designed to stoke enthusiasm, provide potent strategies and accelerate you towards your fitness peaks. Purchase this report, dive into the exhilarating world of HIIT, and supercharge your workout routine like never before. Let's redefine fitness together—Rev it up with HIIT!

Chapter 2. Understanding High-Intensity Interval Training (HIIT)

High-Intensity Interval Training, commonly known as HIIT, is a revolutionary approach that helps individuals harness their fitness potential through concise and intensive exercise bouts. This dynamic exercise regimen has shattered the myth that prolonged periods of activity are necessary for substantial fitness improvements. Science and numerous anecdotes have found that HIIT stimulates remarkable athletic enhancements, boosts metabolic activity, and nurtures holistic health.

2.1. What is High-Intensity Interval Training (HIIT)?

HIIT is a form of cardiovascular exercise strategy alternating short periods of intense anaerobic exercise with less intense recovery periods. This energetic interchanging between high-intensity bouts and brief recovery breaks makes HIIT an incredibly time-efficient way to exercise.

Scientifically, a typical HIIT session involves a warm-up period, then several repetitions of high-intensity exercises separated by medium-intensity exercises for recovery, finally ending with a cool-down period. The high-intensity exercise should be performed at near maximum intensity. The medium exercise should be about 50% intensity. The number of repetitions and length of each depends on the exercise, but may be as little as three repetitions with just 20 seconds of intense exercise.

2.2. The Underlying Science of HIIT

Underpinning every HIIT workout is a solid foundation of science. The effectiveness of HIIT lies in its ability to keep your heart rate up and burn more fat in less time than traditional workout methods. When you engage in a high-intensity interval, it drives your body's repair cycle into hyperdrive, resulting in a higher calorie burn than traditional workouts, even after the workout is complete.

The science supporting HIIT's effectiveness revolves around Excess Post-exercise Oxygen Consumption (EPOC), also known as the "afterburn effect". After a HIIT workout, your oxygen consumption and calorie burning continue at an elevated rate as your body works to restore itself to its resting state. The result? Your metabolism remains revved up, even hours post-workout.

2.3. HIIT Workout Structure

A typical HIIT workout begins with a warm-up phase, followed by intense bouts of exercise interspersed with less-intense recovery phases, and ends with a cooldown. The intense bouts push one's heart and muscles to their limits, creating a demand for oxygen that outstrips the body's ability to deliver — forcing the body into an oxygen debt, paving the way for EPOC.

Each HIIT sequence varies in timing. You might sprint for 30 seconds and then walk for a minute, and repeat. Alternatively, you could engage in a more challenging 2-minute high-intensity burst, followed by a 1-minute recovery. The goal is to continually alternate between high-intensity and recovery periods to keep your heart rate fluctuating.

2.4. Benefits of HIIT

HIIT boasts several benefits that encompass not only physical fitness and weight loss but also cardiorespiratory health and well-being.

1. Efficient and Time-saving: HIIT workouts can be squeezed into busy schedules due to their time-efficient nature. A typical workout can range between 10 to 30 minutes, making them ideal for those struggling to maintain a regular gym routine.

2. Enhanced Calorie Burn: As your heart rate stays elevated throughout a HIIT workout, the calorie burn is significantly higher than conventional workouts.

3. Boosted Metabolic Rate: The metabolic boost associated with HIIT doesn't end with your workout. Increased EPOC means you continue to burn calories at a higher rate, long after you've finished exercising.

4. Improved Cardiovascular and Respiratory Health: Regular practice of HIIT workouts can improve your heart health and lung capacity, improving stamina and overall fitness.

5. No Equipment Necessary: Many HIIT workouts require no special equipment, making it a highly accessible form of exercise for individuals of all backgrounds and fitness levels.

2.5. Designing a HIIT Routine

Designing a HIIT regimen aligns with your individual needs and abilities begins with understanding your current fitness level. Start slow and gradually increase the intensity. Incorporate a mix of exercises like jump squats, burpees, mountain climbers, etc. Remember, the goal is to alternate between exercises that elevate your heart rate and those that allow you to recover.

While HIIT is highly beneficial, it's critical to remember that rest days are equally important to avoid overtraining and burnout. As a rule of thumb, aim for 1-2 HIIT sessions a week, interspersing them with regular, low-impact workouts.

Evolving your fitness regimes with HIIT can be an incredibly rewarding, albeit challenging journey. However, with the right guidance, consistency, and approach, the rewards are plentiful in terms of robust health, peak fitness, and mental wellbeing.

Chapter 3. The Science Behind HIIT: Efficiency Meets Exercise

This revved-up fitness regimen, also known as High-Intensity Interval Training (HIIT), has proven its efficiency by combining vigorous exercises with periods of rest or less-intense activity. The unique structure of this workout style has afforded it scientific recognition and a fast-growing popularity among fitness enthusiasts worldwide.

3.1. Unraveling the Mechanics of HIIT

Let's delve into the core mechanics of HIIT to better understand why it is so beneficial. It revolves around periods of high-intensity exercises interspersed with either complete rest or low-intensity activity. The rationale behind this structure is to recover during rest periods while maintaining an increased heart rate sufficiently to maintain fat burn and muscle stimulation.

Traditional workouts typically involve performing exercises at a constant pace for an extended time. For instance, it might be running or cycling at a continuous speed for about 30 to 60 minutes. HIIT, on the other hand, would involve alternating these exercises—fast sprinting for one minute, then walking or light jogging for two minutes. Importantly, the periods of high-intensity should be near maximal effort, and the rest or lower-intensity periods are merely there to prepare you for the next burst.

3.2. The Energy Systems: ATP and the Role of HIIT

The intensity of an exercise will determine which energy system the body uses. During high-intensity workouts, the body uses the anaerobic energy system, which does not require oxygen, to create adenosine triphosphate (ATP), the cell's main energy source. Lower-intensity exercises rely on the aerobic system, which utilizes oxygen to produce ATP.

During a HIIT workout, the body primary resorts to the anaerobic energy system due to the high-intensity periods. It's this system that facilitates quick bursts of energy for short durations. Post anaerobic activity, the body experiences an oxygen debt, leading to a state called Excess Post-Exercise Oxygen Consumption (EPOC), allowing calories to burn even after the workout is over, enhancing the overall fat-burning potential of HIIT.

3.3. EPOC: The Afterburn Effect

One of the most distinctive features of HIIT is EPOC or the Afterburn effect, a phenomenon otherwise known as the "oxygen deficit." Immediately after an intense workout, your body goes into an EPOC state, which means it continues to consume oxygen at a rate higher than the baseline. This occurs due to various bodily processes like lactate removal, body temperature regulation, and the restoration of energy for muscle contractions.

This increased metabolic rate means that you continue burning calories post-exercise – even at rest – effectively accelerating weight loss and overall caloric expenditure. This effect is particularly pronounced in HIIT due to the intense bursts of exercise that cause a greater disturbance in your body's homeostasis, leading to a more prolonged EPOC period.

3.4. Short Duration, Immense Benefits

One of the key attractions of HIIT is the shorter workout duration. As per the American College of Sports Medicine, a typical HIIT session can range from 20 to 60 minutes. This approach is often more feasible for individuals with a demanding schedule seeking an efficient way to achieve their fitness goals. Despite the shorter duration, HIIT can yield significant fitness improvements due to its intense nature and afterburn effect.

3.5. Cardiovascular Improvements

Multiple studies have shown that HIIT can enhance cardiovascular health. It can reduce heart rate and blood pressure in overweight and obese individuals, usually more than moderate-intensity continuous training (MICT). In fact, HIIT has been found, in some instances, to mitigate the arterial stiffness, which is often associated with cardiovascular risk.

3.6. Muscular Adaptations and Fat Loss

HIIT workouts provoke a high level of muscular effort and adaptation. This effort pushes the body to stimulate mitochondrial biogenesis—increasing the size and number of mitochondria in your muscle cells. As a result, the body's capacity to use oxygen improves, thereby enhancing endurance and total work capacity.

In addition, the high-intensity nature of the workout forces the body to tap into fat stores for energy during rest periods, leading to more significant fat loss. This effect, coupled lwith the EPOC phenomenon, is why HIIT ultimately burns more fat and promotes a lean physique more rapidly compared to traditional workouts.

Our journey into the science behind HIIT reveals an ingenious fusion of efficiency and exercise offering an array of health benefits. Such remarkable efficiency of HIIT has made it not just a fitness fad but an evidence-based approach to achieving and maintaining optimal health. Evidently, the science behind HIIT is increasingly inserting itself into workout routines across the globe, and its success is a testament to its effectiveness. Whatever your fitness goals may be - losing weight, enhancing cardiovascular health, or simply becoming stronger - HIIT provides a formidable tool to conquer those aims in record time.

Chapter 4. Gear Up: Essential Equipment for HIIT

High-Intensity Interval Training (HIIT), as the name suggests, is an intense form of fitness regimen that demands considerable physical activity. Certain specialized equipment can enhance the performance and benefits of your HIIT workouts by providing increased resistance, monitoring your progress, or helping you to target specific muscles. Let's delve into the essential equipment to gear up for HIIT.

4.1. Resistance Bands

Resistance bands are a versatile and inexpensive piece of equipment that can enhance any HIIT workout. They come in a variety of resistance levels, allowing you to gradually increase the difficulty of your exercises as your strength improves. These bands can supplement bodyweight exercises, challenge your muscles under tension, and improve overall strength and mobility.

To incorporate resistance bands into your HIIT, choose bands of appropriate resistance that challenge you but do not compromise your form. Ensure they are not fraying or close to breakage before use. Handle with care, cleaning, drying, and storing them properly to prolong their lifespan.

4.2. Dumbbells

Dumbbells are a classic and crucial piece of gym equipment. They belong in your HIIT arsenal due to their convenience and ease of use. Whether you're performing squat presses, lunges, or deadlifts, dumbbells easily intensify these workout routines.

The recommended starting weight varies depending on each individual's fitness level. Lighter weights (approximately 1-3kg) are ideal for beginners, whereas more accomplished athletes can start with heavier dumbbells. Always pick weights that challenge you slightly, keeping in mind that maintaining form is more crucial than lifting heavy.

4.3. Kettlebells

Kettlebells offer a different dynamic to basic strength training. Their unique shape offers an array of innovative exercises that work muscles from different angles, improving overall functional strength. Kettlebell swings, snatches, and goblet squats are some excellent exercises to consider for a HIIT workout.

Much like dumbbells, kettlebell weight should not compromise your movement techniques. Start with a weight comfortable enough to handle with proper technique, and then continue to raise the weight as your strength and endurance improve.

4.4. Medicine Balls

Medicine balls – or med balls, for short – are an excellent tool for adding an extra difficulty layer to your HIIT sessions. They can be used for a variety of muscle-strengthening exercises such as wall balls, Russian twists, or even a simpler pass-and-catch exercise.

The weight of the medicine ball should ideally sit in a range that you can control sufficiently without difficulty. For beginners, lighter balls (approximately 2-4kg) are advisable. On the other hand, someone well-versed in fitness exercises can go for balls weighing between 6kg and 12kg.

4.5. Heart-Rate Monitor

A heart-rate monitor is not fitness equipment in the traditional sense, but it is a vital tool for tracking your HIIT workouts. This device keeps track of your heart's beats per minute (bpm), offering you a real-time snapshot of your intensity levels.

A heart-rate monitor helps ensure your high-intensity intervals indeed push your heart rate upward of 80% of your maximum heart rate. Simultaneously, during your recovery intervals, it should decrease to around 40-50%. Keeping these percentages in mind, this device plays a pivotal role in ensuring the efficacy of your HIIT workouts. Many come with additional features that track indoor and outdoor workouts, and some even provide sleep analytics.

4.6. Workout Mat

Last but not least, a good quality workout mat is just as important as any other equipment on this list. A good mat creates a soft surface that can protect your joints during high-impact movements and offer a gripping surface for stability. For HIIT workouts, rubber exercise mats are typically preferred due to their durability and the cushioning they provide.

In conclusion, using the right equipment can maximize your HIIT workout effectiveness, improve muscular strength, increase stamina, and inevitably, accelerate your journey towards your fitness peak. Invest in equipment that aligns with your training needs and preferences, and remember that progress comes with consistency and incremental challenges. Happy training!

Remember, it's not about having a plethora of equipment or using the heaviest weights available but maintaining a disciplined regular regimen, challenging your abilities, and gradually elevating your thresholds while working out safely. The equipment is there to assist and enhance. Embark on your HIIT journey with the right gear, determination in your heart, sweat on your brow, and the resolve to become fitter and healthier each day.

Chapter 5. Designing Your HIIT Workout: A Step-by-Step Guide

High-intensity interval training (HIIT) is an incredibly effective exercise regimen that condenses the benefits of prolonged, moderate exercise into a shorter, more intense workout. To ensure that you reap the benefits of HIIT, understanding how to design a custom program suited to your physical needs and goals is essential. Now, let's embark on a methodical journey to design your HIIT workout routine.

5.1. Analyze Your Fitness Level

Before leaping into the HIIT world, it's vital to honestly determine your fitness level. Document a baseline of your current capabilities in terms of strength, endurance, flexibility, and cardio health. This will help you design an effective, safe, and enjoyable program.

To gauge these metrics, you can perform exercises such as:

- Maximum push-ups in a minute: To measure muscle strength and endurance.

- Heart rate post a 10-minute light jog or brisk walk: To provide a basic understanding of cardiovascular health.

- Distance reached by holding a forward bend: This will shed light on flexibility.

- Most importantly, consider talking to a healthcare professional or a certified trainer for an in-depth fitness appraisal.

Dedicate this initial journey to comprehending where you are - it's the platform on which your HIIT workout will be designed.

5.2. Define Your Goals

Next, outline your fitness goals. Are you aiming to lose weight, improve cardio health, build muscle, or increase flexibility? Defining goals empowers the design process by providing direction to the workout specifics—exercise selection, intensity, duration, and so on.

5.3. Choose Exercises

Once your goal is fixed, start to populate your workout with exercises. HIIT is incredibly versatile, compatible with a wide array of exercise types—running, cycling, bodyweight exercises, or even swimming.

Choose exercises aligned with your fitness goals and baseline physical abilities. For instance, a beginner wanting to build strength might include bodyweight exercises like squats, push-ups, or lunges in their HIIT routine.

Ensure that the chosen exercises engage a variety of muscle groups for a wholesome workout.

5.4. Decide On Work and Rest Intervals

The crux of HIIT lies in its intervals—the periods of intense exercise (work) followed by rest or lower-intensity exercise. Initially, starting with a 1:2 work-to-rest ratio (like 30 seconds of high-intensity work followed by 60 seconds of rest) can be useful.

Over time, as your fitness level improves, aim to progress towards a ratio of 1:1 or even greater intensities. However, be careful to adjust these ratios as per your body's feedback.

5.5. Create Your Workout

Once the exercises, work and rest intervals are set, it's time to combine them. Aim for a workout duration of about 15-30 minutes, including warm-up and cool-down periods.

An example HIIT workout could be:

1. Work: 30 seconds intense sprint

2. Rest: 60 seconds brisk walk

3. Repeat: 10 times

Alternately, a bodyweight circuit could also be designed.

5.6. Warm-up and Cool-down

Every HIIT session should begin with a warm-up and end with a cool-down. A warm-up prepares the body for impending exertion, while a cool-down helps the body relax post-workout, reduces muscle soreness, and aids recovery.

5.7. Stay Consistent

Consistency is paramount when it comes to fitness results. Design your program to be sustainable, ensuring you can stick to the regimen long term.

5.8. Measure Progress

Keep track of your progress longitudinally. Notes about workout intensity, endurance, heart rate, and strength will help modify your strategy as you evolve and your fitness level enhances.

Designing a HIIT workout requires thoughtful deliberation about current fitness levels, fitness goals, and personal preferences. The steps provided above serve as a blueprint to tailor-make your HIIT regimen. With this guide, you now stand equipped with knowledge and strategy—both vital in maximizing the effectiveness of your HIIT workouts. Remember to keep workouts challenging, maintain consistency, and above all, enjoy the process. The journey towards peak fitness is as fulfilling as the destination.

HIIT transforms not only your body, but also your mindset—start your transformative journey today!

Chapter 6. Sprinting Ahead: HIIT for Cardio

In the realm of cardiovascular training, High-Intensity Interval Training, or HIIT, has become an exciting alternative to traditional forms of exercise. Unlike steady-state cardio, where you maintain a steady heart rate for an extended period, HIIT workouts are characterized by short, intense periods of exercise, followed by brief recovery periods. This creates a unique dynamic that can lead to substantial cardiovascular benefits in less time.

6.1. The Building Blocks of HIIT Cardio

The core concept behind HIIT is relatively straightforward. First, you need to engage in an activity—like running, cycling, or swimming—at a very high intensity. This is typically done at 80%–90% of your maximum heart rate. After maintaining this intensity for a brief period, typically 30 seconds to a minute, you then slow down and recover at a lower intensity for a similar or slightly longer duration.

It's the contrast between high-intensity work and low-intensity recovery that defines a HIIT workout. The elevated heart rate during the high-intensity bouts stimulates adaptations in your cardiovascular system, increasing your aerobic capacity and improving your overall health and fitness levels.

6.2. Getting Started with HIIT Cardio

Embarking on a HIIT journey begins with a basic understanding of where your fitness level currently stands. A crucial part of starting

HIIT is understanding your maximum heart rate (MHR). A simple formula to estimate MHR is 220 - your age.

This MHR forms the foundation of all your training. The target intensity during high-intensity intervals is usually 80%-90% MHR, while during recovery periods the heart rate should drop down to around 50-70%.

It's important to warm up before diving into an intense workout. About 5 to 10 minutes of light aerobic exercise, such as brisk walking or slow jogging, primes the body and reduces the risk of injury.

Once you're warmed up, it's time to tackle your first high-intensity interval. You can run, cycle, or perform any other high-intensity workout—but no matter what, the idea is to push yourself hard for a short period.

6.3. A Sample HIIT Cardio Workout

Here's a sample introductory HIIT workout for sprinters:

- Warm-up: Jog slowly for 5-10 minutes.

- High-intensity: Sprint at 80%-90% of your MHR for 30 seconds.

- Recovery: Slow down to a walk or slow jog, dropping your heart rate back to around 50%-70% MHR. Maintain this for 60 seconds.

- Repeat: Do this cycle 8-10 times.

- Cool down: Finish off with 5 minutes of easy walking or jogging.

6.4. Why HIIT for Cardio?

HIIT workouts have gained popularity mainly due to their efficiency, and health benefits.

1. Time-efficiency: With HIIT, you're getting the same

cardiovascular benefits as a longer steady-state session in a fraction of the time. A 30-minute HIIT workout, including warm-up and cool-down, can provide the same cardiovascular gains as a 60-minute moderate-intensity cardio workout.

2. Increased metabolic rate: HIIT workouts stimulate excess post-exercise oxygen consumption (EPOC), also known as the "afterburn" effect. This means your body continues to burn calories at a higher rate even after the workout is finished, leading to increased fat loss.

3. Improved cardiovascular and metabolic health: Studies have shown that HIIT workouts can reduce heart rate and blood pressure in overweight and obese individuals. It also improves insulin sensitivity, which helps in managing blood sugar levels.

6.5. The Precautions and Considerations

Despite the benefits, HIIT workouts are intense and could lead to injury or burnout if not performed correctly or if the body isn't allowed adequate recovery.

1. Always warm up: Preparing the body for intense work is crucial. A good warm-up increases body temperature, loosens up the muscles, and gradually raises heart rate, reducing injury risk.

2. Proper recovery: The recovery time given in HIIT is just as important as the intense bursts. It allows your heart rate to come down, preparing the body for the next workout burst.

3. Progress slowly: It's important not to rush the process. Start with fewer cycles and gradually increase as your body becomes comfortable with the workout.

4. Consult a healthcare professional: Particularly if you have any chronic health conditions or haven't exercised in a while, you should speak to a healthcare professional before starting a HIIT

program.

HIIT for cardio can lead to dramatic health benefits in a relatively short amount of time. With a carefully planned regime, you can sprint your way to a fitter, healthier lifestyle. However, as with any fitness routine, the key is in consistency and gradual progression. Happy training!

Chapter 7. Strength Training with HIIT: A New Paradigm

High-Intensity Interval Training, or HIIT, is widely celebrated for its time efficiency, fat-burning capacity, and adaptability to a range of fitness applications. In the context of strength training, the infusion of HIIT principles creates a new, dynamic frontier. Combining elements of traditional strength training with the intensity and pace of HIIT has the potential to redefine workout regimes worldwide.

When discussing HIIT and strength training, two essential aspects come to light – intensity and volume. HIIT revolves around strenuous effort, punctuated by intervals of rest or light activity, while traditional strength training is defined by the manipulation of volume (repetitions and sets), exercise selection and, importantly, rest intervals and weight. Merging the intensity and rhythmic progression of HIIT with the deliberate, targeted movements of strength training is not just compelling; it's transformative.

7.1. Integrating HIIT and Strength Training

Balancing intensity, rest, and volume is paramount in successful HIIT strength training. Each exercise should push the boundaries of exertion, followed by adequate rest to recover and preserve form over subsequent sets. Volume needs to strike a delicate balance – too much, and risk of injury escalates; too little, and results may stagnate.

A popular structure to follow is the 'Tabata Protocol', which outlines a cycle of 20 seconds of high-intensity effort, followed by 10 seconds of rest, continuously repeated for four minutes. This protocol can be applied to exercises like deadlifts or bench presses to bring that high-intensity element into strength training.

However, modifying strength training movements to fit a HIIT format involves careful attention to detail. For example, when performing lifts during the intense interval, the technique should not be compromised. If form begins to waver due to fatigue, the intensity should be reduced or the exercise modified.

Appropriate warm-ups and cool-downs are also crucial, just as with any exercise program. Dynamic warm-ups help prepare the body, while cool-downs with light, static stretching aid recovery.

7.2. Working with Different Muscle Groups

HIIT Strength training provides an excellent platform for compound movements, engaging multiple muscle groups simultaneously and effectively. However, while integrating HIIT and strength workouts, the division of muscle groups demands consideration.

A workable approach could involve designating specific days for different group workouts, like 'push' exercises one day (bench press, overhead press, squat), and 'pull' exercises the next (deadlift, bent-over row, pull-ups). This division allows adequate rest intervals for each muscle group and maintains a high overall intensity of training.

For seasoned workout enthusiasts, advanced techniques like supersets (performing two exercises back-to-back with no rest in between) could be employed. Pairing exercises antagonistically (working opposing muscle groups, e.g., bicep curls and triceps pushdowns) can amplify the benefits while ensuring balanced muscle development.

7.3. Progress Tracking

With the dynamic fusion of HIIT and strength training, it's vital to monitor your progress. Recording your workouts, including exercises, weights used, and reps accomplished, can provide crucial data for analysing improvement and modifying future sessions. Observing the body's response to different intensity levels and adjustments can additionally highlight personal aptitudes and areas for concentration.

7.4. Injuries and Safety Considerations

Like any fitness regimen, potential for injury in HIIT strength training makes caution and safety paramount. Never sacrifice form for intensity. Ensure you master basic lifting techniques before incorporating them into an intense HIIT schedule, and always practice exercises at a lower intensity or weight before jumping to full capacity.

The rest intervals are integral to reducing risk and enhancing the effectiveness of workouts – use them wisely. Additionally, listening to your body goes a long way in injury prevention. Having an occasional easy day or taking a break when needed is essential for any effective fitness regimen, more so in a regimen that's as demanding as HIIT.

In conclusion, the hybrid paradigm of HIIT and strength training opens new horizons of physical fitness. The intensity, rhythm and potent combination of movements promise a robust and efficient workout experience. With informed integration, progress tracking, and attention to safety, this regimen can redefine traditional norms and accelerate fitness gains to breathtaking peaks. However, always remember to consult a professional before radically changing your workouts or attempting any new regimen for the first time.

Chapter 8. Embracing the Burn: Safety Measures and Injury Prevention

High-intensity interval training (HIIT), with its quick bursts of intense exercise interspersed with short rest periods, embodies the spirit of 'no pain, no gain'. But this by no means suggests straining your body recklessly. When combined with proactive safety measures, you can maximise the effectiveness of your HIIT workouts while also reducing the risk of injury.

Safety in HIIT begins with a proper understanding of the body's responses and limitations and continues with the implementation of appropriate measures before, during, and after every workout.

8.1. Understanding Your Body

HIIT is challenging, and it's intended to be. By pushing your body beyond its comfort zone, you stimulate improvements in physical strength and cardiovascular fitness. However, recognizing your personal limits is crucial for avoiding potential harm.

Know the difference between healthy exertion and harmful overexertion. Remember that pain isn't just discomfort—it's the body's warning signal. Pain in the chest, severe breathlessness, or feeling faint should not be ignored. It's a sign to slow down or stop altogether.

The ability to self-monitor your body's response to exertion is invaluable. Listen to your body. Be aware of your perceived exertion and know when to step down the intensity.

8.2. Warm-Up and Cool-Down

HIIT pushes the body hard. Warming up elevates body temperature, increases blood flow to muscles, and reduces the chance of injury, preparing your body for the upcoming rigorous workout. Five to ten minutes of cardio training (like light jogging or stationary cycling) is advisable.

Similarly, cooling down after HIIT aims to gradually reduce heart rate and calm the body. Stretching and light, low-impact activities such as walking can serve as effective cool-down exercises. This not only aids recovery but also helps alleviate post-workout soreness and stiffness.

8.3. Focusing on Form

Focus on form before intensity. It's common for beginners to prioritize speed over correct posture. Performing exercises quickly with incorrect form may lead to severe injuries. Thus, take the time to master the form of each exercise before adding speed and intensity.

8.4. Proper Hydration and Nutrition

With HIIT's high energy demands, regular hydration and proper nutrition are essential. Hydrate throughout the day, not just during workouts. HIIT can cause considerable water loss through sweat, making hydration crucial to replenish lost fluids and maintain endurance.

Nutrition is equally important. Aim for a balanced meal with a mix of protein and complex carbohydrates before and after HIIT to provide energy and assist recovery. Consuming adequate protein aids in muscle repair, and carbohydrates replenish lost energy stores.

8.5. Adapting Workouts and Respecting Rest Days

Everyone has different fitness levels, so modify exercises to match your capacity. Beginners should start with less strenuous routines or add extra rest periods between intervals.

Rest days are vital for heart health and muscle recovery. Include at least two rest days per week in your regimen. Overexertion without sufficient rest can lead to overtraining syndrome, characterized by reduced performance, fatigue, and weakened immunity.

8.6. Common Injuries and How to Prevent Them

HIIT can potentially lead to overuse injuries, including stress fractures, tendinitis, and shin splints. Counteract these risks with diverse workouts that don't put repeated pressure on the same muscle groups and joints.

Let's discuss some common injuries:

- **Sprains and Strains:** Caused by excessive pressures on the joints and muscles. Proper warm-up, focusing on form, and not overloading the weights will substantially reduce the risk.

- **Knee Injuries:** Wrong landing form during plyometric exercises (jumping exercises) often leads to knee injuries. Landing softly, with knees slightly bent, can prevent such injuries.

- **Muscle Pulls:** These can be prevented by not pushing too hard, and by taking adequate rest and recovery time post-workout.

Use safety gear like knee supports, wrist wraps, and proper athletic shoes to additionally reduce the risk of injury.

8.7. Rehabilitation & Recovery

In case of injury, stop all HIIT routines immediately, and seek professional help. Rest, ice, compression, and elevation (RICE) are first aid measures to take while you seek consultation.

HIIT, with all its benefits, demands an equivalent emphasis on care. This chapter has provided the insights needed to approach your workouts safely and effectively. Regular check-ins with your health, adherence to warm-up and cool-down practices, nutritional balance, respect for rest days, and injury preventive measures stand as the pillars of safe HIIT workouts. Arm yourself with these strategies, and you are all set to embrace the burn responsibly.

Chapter 9. HIIT for Different Fitness Levels: Tailoring Your Workout

High-Intensity Interval Training (HIIT) is a versatile method of exercise that can be tailored to benefit fitness enthusiasts of all levels. Whether you're a beginner, an intermediate exerciser, an advanced athlete, a senior, or someone recovering from an injury, HIIT, when adjusted to your needs, can catapult you towards your fitness goals.

9.1. Beginners: Starting Your HIIT Journey

Starting your journey with HIIT as a beginner can be quite exciting yet daunting. Consider the following steps to ease your transition into this highly effective workout regime:

1. **Familiarize Yourself**: Learn about different types of HIIT workouts, the technique's specifics, and required equipment. Understanding the exercises ahead of time ensures safety and efficiency in your training.

2. **Each Effort Counts**: Start with short, intense efforts followed by longer periods of rest or low-intensity exercise. For instance, sprint hard for 20 seconds, then walk or lightly jog for 60 seconds.

3. **Seek Professional Guidance**: Consider enlisting the support of a fitness professional. They can offer guidance, assist with correct form, and keep you motivated.

4. **Listen to Your Body**: This can't be stressed enough. Use perceived exertion and how you feel as a guide to how hard you're working. If you are feeling unusually exhausted, it may be

a sign you should lighten up a bit.

5. **Changing Things Up**: As you get stronger and your body adapts to the workouts, increase the length of your high-intensity intervals.

9.2. Intermediate: Leveling Up Your HIIT Performance

For intermediate exercisers, HIIT offers an exceptional way to level up your fitness performance. Here are ways to spice up your HIIT strategy:

1. **Intensify the Intervals**: Increase the length of your high-intensity periods. This could mean going from 30 seconds of effort to 40 or 45 seconds.

2. **Decrease Rest Duration**: Shrink your rest time in between intervals to keep your heart rate high.

3. **Add Resistance**: Incorporate weighted exercises into your HIIT sessions to build strength alongside endurance.

4. **Vary Your Workouts**: Keeping your body guessing is key to continued progress. Variety will help prevent plateaus and keep your workouts enjoyable.

9.3. Advanced: Optimizing HIIT for Peak Fitness

For advanced athletes, HIIT can be a tool for achieving peak fitness. Consider these strategies when incorporating HIIT into your routine:

1. **Maximize Intensity**: Crank up intensity to ensure you're pushing your limits. This will drive your heart and lungs to their maximum capacity.

2. **Variable Interval Training**: Changing up the lengths of your HIIT intervals can bring about different benefits. Traditional HIIT is great, but throwing in workouts where high-intensity bursts vary from 20 seconds to two minutes adds an extra challenge.

3. **Combination Workouts**: Combine HIIT with other forms of training for all-encompassing fitness benefits. A great example is mixing HIIT with weightlifting.

9.4. Seniors and Injury Recuperation: HIIT Adaptations

Seniors or those in injury recovery can significantly benefit from HIIT, too. Here's how to adapt this routine for these unique conditions:

1. **Check With Health Professionals**: Always get the clearance of healthcare professionals before starting or altering an exercise plan.

2. **Modify the Intensity**: High intensity for a senior or someone recovering could be significantly slower than for a healthy, young adult. Always work at an intensity that feels challenging but manageable.

3. **Choose Low-Impact**: High-impact exercises can increase the risk of injury. Opt for low-impact HIIT options like cycling, swimming, or rowing instead.

4. **Ensure Correct Warm-Up and Cool-Down**: More than others, this cadre of exercisers should pay extra attention to warming up adequately before the workout and cooling down afterwards, to avoid unnecessary injuries.

HIIT is a powerful workout strategy. By adjusting your work-to-rest periods and exercise selection based on your current fitness level, you can safely ramp up your training intensity and see substantial improvements in your overall fitness. With regular HIIT workouts, you can expect an increase in your cardiovascular fitness, muscular strength and endurance, metabolic function, and much more. Whether you're a rookie or a seasoned athlete, there's a version of HIIT that can help fast-track your fitness dreams into reality.

Chapter 10. Fueling HIIT: Nutritional Guidelines

Just as fuel is critical for the smooth running of a vehicle, nutrition plays a pivotal role in the effectiveness of a HIIT routine. A well-designed, holistic nutritional approach can enhance your performance and aid recovery, setting the foundations for long-term results.

10.1. Understanding the Body's Fuel Use

During exercise, our body makes energy using two primary methods - aerobic and anaerobic processes. The choice between these fuel sources depends on the intensity and duration of the physical activity.

Low-intensity and longer-duration exercises mainly rely on aerobic metabolism, burning fat for fuel. On the other hand, high-intensity, short-duration workouts like HIIT predominantly tap into the anaerobic energy pathway, utilizing carbohydrates stored in muscles. However, both fats and carbohydrates fuel exercise at all intensities, with the mix changing depending on intensity.

10.2. Fueling Before a HIIT Workout

Timing and choosing the correct pre-workout meals can help optimize your body's fuel utilization during the workout.

1. Carbohydrates: Consume a meal or snack rich in complex carbohydrates 1-2 hours before beginning your HIIT session. Foods such as brown rice, oats, whole grain bread, and bananas provide slow-releasing energy, preparing your body for the high-

intensity workout. Avoid consuming high-fiber foods or excessive protein close to your workout as it may cause digestive discomfort.

2. Proteins: Include a moderate amount of protein in your pre-workout to help minimize muscle protein breakdown during the exercise.

3. Hydration: Begin your workouts well-hydrated. Dehydration can compromise your body's efficiency and resultant output, negatively impacting workout performance.

10.3. Fueling During a HIIT Workout

Since HIIT workouts are short, often under 30 minutes, there's generally no need to eat or drink other than water during the session. However, if your session lasts longer than an hour, a small carbohydrate-rich snack or sports drink can help maintain energy levels.

10.4. Fueling After a HIIT Workout

Post-workout nutrition is critical for recovery and muscle protein synthesis. It's a golden window to refuel expended glycogen stores and provide essential amino acids to the muscles.

1. Carbohydrates: Post-exercise, your body needs carbohydrates to replenish the diminished glycogen stores. Opt for meals or snacks that include high-quality, complex carbohydrates.

2. Proteins: Consuming protein post-HIIT aids in muscle repair and growth. Incorporate easily digestible, high-quality proteins in your post-workout meal to supply essential amino acids to your muscles.

3. Hydration: Rehydrate post-exercise to replace the fluids lost through sweat. You can also opt for rehydration drinks

containing electrolytes which are lost during intense sessions.

10.5. Sample Meals

Here are a few examples of meals and snacks that can be built into HIIT nutritional regimens.

- Pre-workout Meal: A bowl of oatmeal topped with a small handful of nuts (e.g., almonds or walnuts), some fruits (e.g., berries or banana slices), and a sprinkle of seeds (chia or flax seeds).

- Pre-workout Snack (if needed): A slice of whole-grain toast with a smear of almond butter.

- Post-workout Meal: Grilled chicken, steamed broccoli, and quinoa. Vegetarians/Vegans can replace chicken with a protein-packed plant-based alternative such as tofu or tempeh.

- Post-workout Snack: A protein shake made with protein powder, a banana, and a handful of spinach, blended with almond milk.

Remember, hydration plays a significant role in your performance, so drink plenty of water throughout the day, not just during or after the workout.

10.6. Supplements and HIIT

Research shows that certain nutritional supplements can complement your HIIT sessions. Creatine enhances high-intensity exercise capacity and lean body mass gain. Beta-alanine can also improve exercise performance, while protein supplements support muscle protein synthesis and recovery.

However, note that supplements should not replace a well-balanced diet but rather work synergistically with it. Seek professional advice before introducing any supplements into your regimen.

10.7. Listen to Your Body

Finally, remember that nutritional needs vary from person to person and can be impacted by factors like age, gender, size, and individual metabolic rates. The guidelines above are meant to serve as a starting point. Listen to your body, and adjust your nutritional approach as necessary.

Uplifting your nutritional game is the key to maximizing HIIT benefits. Once fine-tuned, your well-fed physiology partners with this distinct, powerful workout program, to deliver results in record time. Eating right is your gateway to stronger, faster, leaner, and healthier—it's your fuel for the HIIT revolution.

Chapter 11. Real Life Success Stories: Inspirational HIIT Journeys

Here are some stories about people who discovered the potent potential of High-Intensity Interval Training (HIIT) and became fitter, healthier, and happier. Behind every success story, there is a journey filled with moments of struggle, determination, perseverance, and, eventually, achievement. Let's immerse ourselves in these inspirational tales.

11.1. The Tale Of John: Office Worker To Fitness Standout

John was a dedicated office worker, regularly clocking in 10-hour days with little room for exercise. His sedentary lifestyle led to weight gain, lowered energy levels, and a constant feeling of lethargy. One day, he stumbled upon a blog about HIIT, and it triggered a desire for change.

John carved out half an hour every weekday morning and started with 30-second intervals of high-intensity exercises, followed by one-minute rest periods. Soon, he noticed a increase in his energy levels and started seeing physical changes. Despite having a tight schedule, HIIT allowed John to achieve his fitness goals without disrupting his work commitments.

11.2. Annie's Pursuit Of Post-Pregnancy Fitness

Annie, a young mother, was juggling the demands of infant care, housework, and her own postnatal health. Despite her desire to regain her pre-pregnancy fitness, lengthy workouts were not feasible. Her doctor suggested giving HIIT a try.

She began with short bursts of intense exercises during her baby's nap times. She would work as hard as she could for 20 seconds, then take a 10-second rest before repeating the cycle. As she grew stronger, Annie diversified her workouts, adding elements like burpees, mountain climbers, and high knees. Within six months, she was back to her pre-pregnancy fitness level.

11.3. George's Turnaround: Combatting Commoditized Fitness Routines

Meet George, a fitness enthusiast stuck in a monotonous cycle of conventional workouts. Long periods of cardio and weightlifting spurred initial gains, but soon he hit a plateau. Frustrated by his stagnation, he was introduced to HIIT by a friend.

Incorporating HIIT circuits after his regular workout immediately brought a new challenge. George began experiencing visible improvements in his muscular endurance and overall strength. Furthermore, he appreciated the variety HIIT brought to his routine. His fitness journey transformed from a monotonous chore into an engaging habit.

11.4. Rachel: Tackling Aging Gracefully

At 60, Rachel was seeking an exercise routine to mitigate the effects of aging and ensure she remained active and independent. Her physiotherapist recommended HIIT, emphasizing its effectiveness and efficiency.

Initially, Rachel was sceptical and worried it would be too challenging. However, by modifying the exercises to suit her physical capabilities and slowly increasing intensity, Rachel not only coped with HIIT but also started enjoying the sessions. Today, she boasts more robust cardiovascular health, confirming that age is no bar to adopting HIIT and enjoying its benefits.

11.5. Lucy And The Pursuit Of Athletic Performance

Lucy, a passionate amateur soccer player, realized she needed a fitness edge to perform at her best. After researching various fitness routines, she decided to dedicate a portion of her training to HIIT.

Initially, maintaining intensity was a challenge, but she persisted, eventually improving her performance on the field. HIIT didn't just enhance her endurance but also improved her sprinting and recovery times. Lucy's pursuit of improved athletic performance was met with HIIT, turning her into a valuable asset for her team.

These stories underscore the transformative potential of HIIT. Different age groups, fitness aims, lifestyles, and time commitments—HIIT has proven to be an adaptable and efficient solution. It's not just about physical gains; these success stories underline the role of willpower, dedication, and the mental strength HIIT instills, along with physical prowess, to push beyond perceived limits.

On your journey, you may stumble, face setbacks, maybe even hit plateaus. But, remember the journeys of John, Annie, George, Rachel, and Lucy. They too encountered challenges, but their grit and resolve, combined with the dynamism of HIIT, eventually led them to remarkable transformations. Stay patient, stay committed, and embrace HIIT wholeheartedly. Your inspirational HIIT journey could be the next one shared with the world.

www.ingramcontent.com/pod-product-compliance
Lightning Source LLC
Chambersburg PA
CBHW071015260726

48661CB00007B/2982